INTRODUCTION

Lipedema is a chronic and often misunderstood condition characterized by abnormal fat accumulation, typically in the lower limbs, leading to disproportionate and painful swelling. This condition primarily affects women, and its etiology remains under-researched, making diagnosis and effective management challenging. Lipedema is not related to obesity or lifestyle factors, and despite its prevalence, it is frequently misdiagnosed or overlooked, contributing to the physical and emotional burdens faced by those affected.

Managing the symptoms of lipedema requires a comprehensive approach that goes beyond traditional weight loss methods. The Relationship of Adipose Distribution (RAD) Diet for Lipedema emerges as a holistic dietary strategy aimed at addressing the unique challenges posed by this condition. This diet emphasizes specific nutritional choices and lifestyle modifications tailored to alleviate symptoms and improve overall well-being for individuals living with lipedema.

The RAD Diet acknowledges the complexities of lipedema, considering factors such as inflammation, lymphatic dysfunction, and hormonal influences on fat distribution.

By incorporating anti-inflammatory foods, promoting lymphatic flow, and addressing hormonal balance through nutrition, the RAD Diet aims to empower individuals with practical tools to better manage the impact of lipedema on their daily lives.

CHAPTER ONE

Definition of Lipedema

Lipedema is a chronic and often underdiagnosed condition characterized by the abnormal and disproportionate accumulation of fat, primarily in the lower extremities, hips, and buttocks. This disorder primarily affects women, although rare cases have been reported in men. Lipedema is distinct from obesity, as it is not a result of excessive calorie intake or a sedentary lifestyle, and individuals with lipedema often experience difficulty losing weight in the affected areas through traditional diet and exercise.

CAUSES AND RISK FACTORS OF LIPEDEMA

Lipedema is a complex and multifaceted condition influenced by a combination of genetic, hormonal, and other factors. Understanding the various elements contributing to the development of lipedema is crucial for accurate diagnosis and the formulation of effective management strategies.

A. Genetic Factors: Genetic predisposition plays a significant role in the development of lipedema. There is a notable familial clustering of the condition, suggesting a hereditary component. Individuals with a family history of lipedema are at an increased risk of experiencing the disorder themselves. While specific genetic markers associated with lipedema are still under investigation, the evidence of familial links underscores the importance of genetic factors in its etiology.

B. Hormonal Influences: Hormonal influences, particularly those related to female reproductive hormones, are believed to contribute to the development and exacerbation of lipedema. The condition predominantly affects women, and hormonal changes associated with puberty, pregnancy, and menopause may trigger or worsen symptoms. Hormones such as estrogen may play a role in fat metabolism and distribution, impacting the adipose tissue characteristic of lipedema. Hormonal fluctuations throughout a woman's life may explain the predominantly female prevalence and the worsening of symptoms during hormonal milestones.

C. Possible Links to Obesity: While lipedema is distinct from obesity, there is an association between the two conditions, leading to potential misdiagnosis or misunderstanding. Lipedema often coexists with obesity, and individuals with lipedema may face challenges in weight management through traditional diet and exercise. The disproportionate fat distribution in lipedema can lead to misconceptions, but it is essential to recognize that lipedema is not a consequence of obesity. Instead, obesity and lipedema may share common pathways, and managing one condition does not necessarily resolve the other.

D. Other Contributing Factors: Several other factors contribute to the development and progression of lipedema. Chronic inflammation is considered a potential contributor, as inflammatory processes can affect adipose tissue and exacerbate symptoms. Additionally, impaired lymphatic function is observed in the later stages of lipedema, suggesting a potential interplay between lymphatic dysfunction and the accumulation of excess fat. Trauma or injury to the affected areas may also trigger or worsen lipedema symptoms.

Environmental factors, such as a sedentary lifestyle and dietary choices, may influence the severity of symptoms, but they are not primary causes of lipedema.

SYMPTOMS OF LIPEDEMA

Lipedema is a chronic condition characterized by distinctive symptoms, primarily involving the abnormal and disproportionate accumulation of fat, typically in the lower extremities. Recognizing the array of symptoms associated with lipedema is crucial for early diagnosis and the development of effective management strategies.

1. Disproportionate Fat Distribution:
    a. A hallmark symptom of lipedema is the abnormal distribution of fat, often presenting as a symmetrical accumulation in the lower limbs, hips, and buttocks. This creates a characteristic "column-like" appearance, with a distinct boundary at the ankles and wrists. Notably, the hands and feet are spared from this excessive fat deposition.
2. Pain and Tenderness:
    a. Individuals with lipedema commonly experience pain and tenderness in the affected areas. This discomfort can range from mild to severe and may be exacerbated by pressure from clothing or prolonged standing.

3. Easy Bruising:
    a. Lipedema-prone fat is more fragile and prone to bruising, even with minimal trauma or pressure, contributing to easy bruising. The bruising can occur spontaneously or as a result of minor injuries.
4. Increased Sensitivity to Touch:
    a. The affected areas may become more sensitive to touch, and individuals with lipedema may find that even light pressure causes discomfort. This heightened sensitivity is often related to the increased pressure within the affected fat compartments.
5. Swelling and Fluid Retention:
    a. Progressive swelling, particularly in the lower limbs, is a common symptom of lipedema. This swelling is not usually associated with pitting (the retention of an indentation after pressure is applied) and can be exacerbated by factors such as heat or prolonged standing.
6. Stages of Progression:
    a. Lipedema typically progresses in stages, with early stages characterized by soft, non-pitting edema and later stages involving increased fibrosis and potential lymphatic impairment. As the condition advances, the skin may take on a "peau d'orange" or orange peel-like appearance.
7. Worsening Symptoms with Hormonal Changes:
    a. Hormonal fluctuations, such as those

occurring during puberty, pregnancy, and menopause, can worsen lipedema symptoms. This suggests a hormonal influence in the development and exacerbation of the condition.

8. Psychological Impact:

    a. Beyond the physical symptoms, lipedema can have a profound psychological impact on individuals. The noticeable changes in body shape may contribute to body image issues, leading to emotional distress and a diminished quality of life.

DIAGNOSIS OF LIPEDEMA

Diagnosing lipedema can be a complex process that requires a thorough assessment of clinical symptoms, medical history, and, in some cases, imaging studies. Given that lipedema is often underdiagnosed or misidentified. The following outlines the key components involved in the diagnosis of lipedema:

1. Clinical Evaluation:
    a. A healthcare professional, often a specialist such as a vascular surgeon, dermatologist, or lymphedema therapist, will conduct a comprehensive clinical evaluation. This involves a thorough examination of the patient's medical history, symptoms, and physical characteristics. Clinicians pay close attention to the distribution of excess fat, the presence of tenderness, bruising tendencies, and any associated pain.
2. Rule Out Other Conditions:
    a. Since lipedema shares similarities with other conditions such as lymphedema, Dercum's disease, and obesity, it is crucial to rule out these potential differential

diagnoses. Specialized tests, imaging studies, and consultations with relevant specialists may be necessary to ensure an accurate diagnosis.

3. Duplex Ultrasound:
   a. Duplex ultrasound is a non-invasive imaging technique that may be used to assess blood flow and rule out vascular conditions. While lipedema is primarily a disorder of fatty tissue, the potential coexistence of venous disorders requires careful examination.

4. MRI (Magnetic Resonance Imaging):
   a. In some cases, magnetic resonance imaging may be employed to visualize adipose tissue distribution, assess the severity of fibrosis, and rule out other conditions. MRI provides detailed images of soft tissues, aiding in the identification of characteristic features of lipedema.

5. Bioimpedance Analysis:
   a. Bioimpedance analysis measures the resistance of electrical flow through tissues, helping assess body fluids' composition. This can be useful in distinguishing lipedema from conditions involving significant fluid retention.

6. Lymphoscintigraphy:
   a. Lymphoscintigraphy is a nuclear medicine imaging technique used to evaluate the lymphatic system. It can be employed to identify any impairment in lymphatic function, which may be

relevant in later stages of lipedema.

7. Hormonal Assessment:
    a. Since hormonal influences are believed to contribute to the development and exacerbation of lipedema, hormonal assessments, particularly of reproductive hormones, may be considered.

8. Patient History and Symptoms:
    a. A detailed patient history is essential, with a focus on the onset and progression of symptoms, hormonal milestones (such as puberty and pregnancy), and any family history of similar conditions. Understanding the psychological impact of lipedema is also crucial in providing comprehensive care.

TREATMENT APPROACHES FOR LIPEDEMA

Lipedema management involves a multidimensional approach that addresses the condition's physical and psychological aspects. Treatment strategies range from conservative measures to surgical interventions, and ongoing research is exploring pharmacological options. Tailoring the approach to the individual's symptoms and stage of lipedema is crucial for optimizing outcomes.

A. Conservative Management:

1. Compression Therapy:
    a. Description: Compression therapy involves the use of compression garments to reduce swelling, support venous and lymphatic function, and alleviate pain.
    b. Effectiveness: Compression garments, such as compression stockings or wraps, can help manage edema and provide symptomatic relief. They should be properly fitted and worn consistently for optimal results.
2. Manual Lymphatic Drainage (MLD):
    a. Description: MLD is a specialized

massage technique designed to stimulate lymphatic flow, reduce swelling, and improve overall lymphatic function.

b. Effectiveness: MLD, when performed by trained therapists, can enhance the drainage of excess fluid and reduce tissue congestion. It is often used in conjunction with compression therapy.

3. Exercise Recommendations:

a. Description: Low-impact exercises, such as swimming, walking, or cycling, are recommended to improve overall cardiovascular health, promote lymphatic flow, and enhance muscle tone.

b. Effectiveness: Regular, gentle exercise can contribute to improved circulation, muscle support, and overall well-being. It is essential to tailor exercise regimens to individual capabilities and progress gradually.

B. Surgical Interventions:

1. Liposuction:

a. Description: Liposuction is a surgical procedure that involves the removal of excess fat deposits from specific areas of the body using suction.

b. Effectiveness: Liposuction is considered an effective and long-lasting intervention for reducing the disproportionate fat deposits associated with lipedema. Water-assisted liposuction and tumescent liposuction are commonly employed techniques.

2. Other Surgical Options:

    a. Description: In advanced cases or when fibrosis is present, surgical procedures such as debulking and excision may be considered to remove excess tissue.

    b. Effectiveness: These procedures aim to reshape the affected areas and improve mobility and overall function. However, they are generally reserved for severe cases and may carry more significant risks.

C. Medications and Pharmacological Approaches:

1. Current Medications:

    a. Description: Currently, no specific medication is approved solely for treating lipedema. However, certain medications, such as anti-inflammatory drugs, may be prescribed to manage associated symptoms like pain and inflammation.

    b. Effectiveness: Medications may offer symptomatic relief but do not address the underlying cause of lipedema.

2. Emerging Treatments:

    a. Description: Ongoing research is exploring potential pharmacological interventions for lipedema, including drugs that target inflammation, adipose tissue metabolism, and hormonal regulation.

    b. Effectiveness: While promising, these

emerging treatments are still in the investigational stages, and further research is needed to establish their safety and efficacy.

COMPLICATIONS OF LIPEDEMA

Lipedema, while primarily characterized by the abnormal accumulation of fat, can lead to various complications that impact both physical and emotional well-being. Understanding and addressing these complications are essential for management and improved quality of life for individuals affected by lipedema.

1. Chronic Pain:
    a. Description: Persistent pain is a common and often debilitating complication of lipedema. The increased pressure within the affected fat compartments and the compression of surrounding structures contribute to chronic discomfort.
2. Limited Mobility:
    a. Description: The disproportionate distribution of fat in the lower extremities can lead to limited mobility and difficulties with ambulation. Reduced mobility may further contribute to a sedentary lifestyle, exacerbating the challenges associated with lipedema.
3. Joint Stress and Osteoarthritis:
    a. Description: The excess weight and

altered biomechanics resulting from lipedema can increase joint stress, potentially leading to premature wear and tear. This may contribute to the development of osteoarthritis in affected joints.

4. Increased Risk of Infections:
    a. Description: The compromised lymphatic flow associated with advanced stages of lipedema can increase the risk of recurrent infections, such as cellulitis. The impaired ability to clear bacteria from the affected areas contributes to this heightened risk.

5. Psychological Impact:
    a. Description: The visible changes in body shape and the challenges associated with living with a chronic condition can lead to psychological complications. Individuals with lipedema may experience body image issues, depression, anxiety, and diminished quality of life.

6. Lymphatic Dysfunction:
    a. Description: In later stages of lipedema, impaired lymphatic function may contribute to the progression of the condition. Lymphedema, characterized by the accumulation of protein-rich fluid, can develop, leading to additional swelling and tissue changes.

7. Complications from Surgical Interventions:
    a. Description: Surgical interventions, such

as liposuction or debulking procedures, carry inherent risks and potential complications. These may include infection, hematoma, scarring, and changes in sensation.

8. Impact on Daily Activities:

    a. Description: The physical symptoms and limitations associated with lipedema can impact daily activities, including self-care, work, and social interactions. Individuals may face challenges in finding suitable clothing, participating in physical activities, and maintaining a regular routine.

9. Financial and Social Burden:

    a. Description: The financial burden of managing lipedema, including the costs associated with compression garments, medical treatments, and potential surgical interventions, can be significant. Additionally, individuals may experience social challenges, including stigma, reduced participation in social events, and feelings of isolation.

CHAPTER TWO

Explanation of the RAD Diet

The Relationship of Adipose Distribution (RAD) Diet is a specialized dietary approach designed to address the unique challenges faced by individuals with lipedema. Lipedema is a chronic condition characterized by abnormal fat accumulation, typically in the lower limbs, hips, and buttocks. The RAD Diet recognizes the multifaceted nature of lipedema, incorporating nutritional strategies to mitigate symptoms and enhance overall well-being. Here are the fundamental principles of the RAD Diet:

1. Inflammation Reduction:
   a. The RAD Diet emphasizes foods with anti-inflammatory properties to address the chronic inflammation associated with lipedema. This includes incorporating fruits, vegetables, fatty fish rich in omega-3 fatty acids and nuts while minimizing the intake of pro-inflammatory foods, such as processed sugars and saturated fats.

2. Lymphatic Support:
   a. Lymphatic dysfunction is joint in advanced stages of lipedema. The RAD Diet promotes foods that support lymphatic function, such as foods rich in antioxidants (berries, leafy

greens), hydrating foods (cucumbers, watermelon), and those with mild diuretic properties (asparagus, celery).

3. Balanced Nutrition:
    a. The RAD Diet emphasizes a balanced and nutrient-dense approach to nutrition. This involves incorporating a variety of foods to ensure adequate intake of essential vitamins, minerals, and macronutrients. Whole grains, lean proteins, healthy fats, and a colorful array of fruits and vegetables form the foundation of this approach.
4. Hormonal Balance:
    a. Hormonal factors play a role in the development and progression of lipedema. The RAD Diet addresses hormonal balance by incorporating foods that support hormone regulation. This includes including sources of healthy fats (avocado, olive oil), fiber-rich foods, and complex carbohydrates to promote stable blood sugar levels.
5. Hydration:
    a. Proper hydration is essential for overall health and can also contribute to lymphatic function. The RAD Diet encourages an adequate intake of water and includes hydrating foods such as water-rich fruits and vegetables.
6. Mindful Eating:
    a. Mindful eating is an integral aspect of the RAD Diet. This involves paying attention

to hunger and fullness cues, savoring each bite, and cultivating a positive relationship with food. Mindful eating can contribute to a healthier approach to meals and address emotional aspects associated with living with lipedema.

7. Individualized Approach:
   a. The RAD Diet recognizes that each person with lipedema is unique, and dietary needs may vary. It encourages individuals to listen to their bodies, make choices that align with their preferences and sensitivities, and work closely with healthcare professionals or dietitians for personalized guidance.

8. Sustainable Lifestyle Changes:
   a. Sustainability is a vital principle of the RAD Diet. Rather than focusing on restrictive measures or short-term solutions, it promotes long-term lifestyle changes that are realistic and manageable. This includes adopting dietary habits that can be sustained over time for ongoing symptom management.

THE IMPORTANCE OF FOLLOWING THE RAD DIET AS A LIPEDEMA PATIENT

Living with lipedema presents unique challenges, and managing the condition requires a multifaceted approach. Adopting the Relationship of Adipose Distribution (RAD) Diet is an integral aspect of this comprehensive strategy. The importance of following the RAD Diet as a lipedema patient cannot be overstated, as it offers a tailored and holistic approach to nutrition that addresses the specific needs and challenges associated with this chronic condition.

1. Inflammation Management:
    a. Lipedema is often accompanied by chronic inflammation, contributing to pain and discomfort. The RAD Diet emphasizes anti-inflammatory foods, such as fruits, vegetables, and omega-3 fatty acids, which may help mitigate inflammation, alleviate symptoms, and improve overall well-being.
2. Lymphatic Support:

    a. Lymphatic dysfunction is a common aspect of advanced lipedema. The RAD Diet incorporates foods that support lymphatic function, such as hydrating fruits and vegetables. Adequate hydration and a diet rich in antioxidants can contribute to maintaining optimal lymphatic flow.

3. Hormonal Balance:

    a. Hormonal factors play a role in the development and progression of lipedema. The RAD Diet includes foods that support hormonal balance, helping to regulate estrogen levels and mitigate the impact of hormonal fluctuations on the condition.

4. Weight Management:

    a. While lipedema is not caused by obesity, the RAD Diet emphasizes a balanced and nutrient-dense approach to nutrition, promoting overall health and potentially supporting weight management. This can be particularly beneficial as excess weight can exacerbate the symptoms associated with lipedema.

5. Mindful Eating for Emotional Well-Being:

    a. The RAD Diet encourages mindful eating, fostering a positive relationship with food. For individuals with lipedema, who may face emotional challenges due to the visible changes in body shape, this aspect of the diet can contribute to improved emotional well-being and a healthier mindset towards nutrition.

6. Individualized Approach:
    a. Every person with lipedema is unique, and the RAD Diet recognizes the importance of individualized approaches to nutrition. Patients can create sustainable habits that align with their specific needs by tailoring dietary choices to personal preferences, sensitivities, and lifestyles.
7. Long-Term Lifestyle Changes:
    a. The RAD Diet is not a short-term fix but rather a lifestyle approach. By adopting sustainable dietary changes, individuals with lipedema can integrate nutritional habits into their daily lives, promoting ongoing symptom management and overall health.

FOODS TO AVOID

Here is the list of foods to avoid when following the RAD Diet for lipedema:

1. Processed Sugars:
    a. Foods high in refined sugars, such as candies, pastries, and sugary beverages, can contribute to inflammation and may lead to fluctuations in blood sugar levels. These should be limited to supporting overall health and managing inflammation.
2. Saturated and Trans Fats:
    a. High amounts of saturated fats, often found in fried foods, processed snacks, and certain cooking oils, can contribute to inflammation. Trans fats, commonly present in some processed foods, margarine, and fried items, should also be avoided.
3. Excessive Salt:
    a. High sodium intake can contribute to fluid retention, exacerbating swelling associated with lipedema. Processed and packaged foods, as well as excessive use of table salt, should be limited.
4. Processed and Packaged Foods:
    a. Processed and packaged foods often

contain additives, preservatives, and artificial ingredients that may contribute to inflammation. These include convenience foods, pre-packaged meals, and snacks with long ingredient lists.

5. Red and Processed Meats:
    a. Red meats, particularly those processed or high in saturated fats, can contribute to inflammation. Limiting the intake of processed meats like sausages, hot dogs, and bacon is advisable.
6. Dairy Products with Hormones:
    a. Some dairy products contain added hormones, which can disrupt hormonal balance. Hormone-free or organic dairy options may be a preferable alternative.
7. Gluten-Containing Grains:
    a. Some individuals with lipedema may have sensitivities to gluten, a protein found in wheat, barley, and rye. Gluten-containing grains may contribute to inflammation for those with gluten sensitivity, and alternatives like gluten-free grains can be considered.
8. Alcohol and Caffeine:
    a. Excessive alcohol and caffeine intake can potentially contribute to inflammation and may impact hormonal balance. Moderation is vital, and individuals should be mindful of how these substances affect their symptoms.
9. Artificial Sweeteners:
    a. Some artificial sweeteners may have

potential health concerns and may not contribute positively to overall well-being. In moderation, natural sweeteners, such as stevia or honey, may be considered alternatives.

10. Highly Processed and Refined Foods:
   a. Highly processed and refined foods, including white bread, white rice, and certain cereals, lack the nutritional benefits found in whole grains. Choosing natural, unprocessed alternatives is encouraged.

SAMPLE MEAL PLAN

Here's a sample RAD Diet meal plan for seven days:

Day 1:

Breakfast:

• Quinoa Breakfast Bowl:

• Cooked Quinoa

• Fresh berries (blueberries, strawberries)

• Chopped nuts (almonds, walnuts)

• Greek yogurt

• Drizzle of honey

Lunch:

• Grilled Chicken Salad:

• Grilled chicken breast

• Mixed greens (spinach, arugula)

• Cherry tomatoes

• Cucumber slices

• Avocado

• Olive oil and lemon dressing

Snack:

• Sliced Apple with Almond Butter:

• Apple slices

- Natural almond butter

Dinner:

- Baked Salmon with Quinoa and Roasted Vegetables:
- Baked salmon fillet
- Quinoa
- Roasted zucchini, cherry tomatoes, and bell peppers
- Fresh lemon wedges

Day 2:

Breakfast:

- Smoothie Bowl:
- Blended mix of mixed berries (blueberries, raspberries)
- Banana
- Greek yogurt
- Topped with chia seeds and sliced kiwi

Lunch:

- Lentil and Vegetable Soup:
- Homemade lentil soup with carrots, celery, and spinach
- Side of whole grain crackers

Snack:

- Greek Yogurt Parfait:
- Greek yogurt
- Layered with sliced peaches and a sprinkle of granola

Dinner:

- Stir-fried tofu with Quinoa:
- Stir-fried tofu with broccoli, bell peppers, and snap peas

- Served over Quinoa
- Drizzled with a light soy-ginger sauce

Day 3:

Breakfast:

- Overnight Oats:
- Rolled oats soaked in almond milk
- Mixed with sliced strawberries, chia seeds, and a touch of honey

Lunch:

- Chickpea Salad:
- Mixed chickpeas
- Cherry tomatoes
- Cucumber
- Red onion
- Feta cheese
- Olive oil and balsamic vinegar dressing

Snack:

- Hummus with Veggie Sticks:
- Carrot and cucumber sticks
- Hummus for dipping

Dinner:

- Grilled Turkey Burgers with Sweet Potato Fries:
- Grilled turkey burgers on whole grain buns
- Baked sweet potato fries
- Side salad with mixed greens and vinaigrette

Day 4:

Breakfast:

• Avocado and Tomato Toast:

• Whole grain toast

• Mashed avocado

• Sliced tomatoes

• Sprinkle of sesame seeds

Lunch:

• Quinoa and Black Bean Bowl:

• Cooked Quinoa

• Black beans

• Corn kernels

• Diced red bell pepper

• Sliced avocado

• Lime-cilantro dressing

Snack:

• Fresh Fruit Salad:

• Watermelon cubes

• Pineapple chunks

• Grapes

• Fresh mint

Dinner:

• Grilled Shrimp with Brown Rice and Asparagus:

• Grilled shrimp skewers

• Brown rice

• Steamed asparagus

• Lemon-garlic butter sauce

Day 5:

Breakfast:

• Chia Seed Pudding:

• Chia seeds soaked in almond milk

• Topped with sliced strawberries and a sprinkle of shredded coconut

Lunch:

• Spinach and Feta Stuffed Bell Peppers:

• Bell peppers stuffed with a mixture of spinach, feta, and Quinoa

• Side of mixed green salad with olive oil dressing

Snack:

• Trail Mix:

• Mixed nuts (almonds, walnuts)

• Dried cranberries

• Dark chocolate pieces

Dinner:

• Baked Cod with Lemon and Herbs:

• Baked cod fillets with a drizzle of olive oil, lemon, and fresh herbs

• Quinoa pilaf with roasted Brussels sprouts

Day 6:

Breakfast:

• Green Smoothie:

- Spinach, kale, and banana blended with almond milk
- Protein powder (optional)
- Chilled for a refreshing start

Lunch:

- Mediterranean Chickpea Salad:
- Chickpeas
- Cherry tomatoes
- Cucumber
- Kalamata olives
- Feta cheese
- Olive oil and lemon dressing

Snack:

- Cottage Cheese with Pineapple:
- Low-fat cottage cheese
- Fresh pineapple chunks

Dinner:

- Grilled Chicken Breast with Quinoa and Roasted Vegetables:
- Grilled chicken breast seasoned with herbs
- Quinoa
- Roasted carrots, broccoli, and red bell peppers

Day 7:

Breakfast:

- Whole Grain Pancakes with Berries:
- Whole grain pancakes topped with mixed berries

- Drizzle of maple syrup

Lunch:

- Turkey and Avocado Wrap:

- Whole grain wrap with turkey slices, avocado, lettuce, and tomato

- Side of cucumber and cherry tomato salad with olive oil dressing

Snack:

- Yogurt with Berries:

- Low-fat yogurt

- Mixed berries (blueberries, raspberries)

Dinner:

- Vegetable Stir-Fry with Tofu:

- Stir-fried broccoli, snap peas, and bell peppers with tofu

- Brown rice

- Light soy-ginger sauce

GROCERY SHOPPING LIST

Preparing for this specialized diet requires a well-thought-out grocery shopping list to ensure you have the right ingredients on hand. Here's a guide for your RAD Diet grocery shopping:

Fresh Produce:

1. Leafy greens (spinach, kale, arugula)
2. Colorful vegetables (bell peppers, carrots, broccoli, asparagus)
3. Avocados
4. Cucumbers
5. Tomatoes
6. Berries (blueberries, strawberries, raspberries)
7. Citrus fruits (lemons, oranges, grapefruits)
8. Apples
9. Kiwi
10. Watermelon
11. Pineapple
12. Fresh herbs (cilantro, mint, basil)

Proteins:

1. Lean poultry (chicken breast, turkey)
2. Fatty fish (salmon, cod)
3. Tofu

4. Greek yogurt (unsweetened)
5. Eggs
6. Legumes (chickpeas, lentils, black beans)

Whole Grains:

1. Quinoa
2. Brown rice
3. Whole grain oats
4. Whole grain bread or wraps
5. Buckwheat flour (for pancakes or alternative baked goods)

Nuts and Seeds:

1. Almonds
2. Walnuts
3. Chia seeds
4. Flaxseeds
5. Sesame seeds

Healthy Fats:

1. Olive oil (extra virgin)
2. Avocado oil
3. Coconut oil
4. Nut butters (almond, peanut, or cashew)

Dairy and Alternatives:

1. Greek yogurt (unsweetened)
2. Cottage cheese
3. Feta cheese
4. Non-dairy milk (almond, coconut, or soy)

Herbs and Spices:

1. Turmeric
2. Ginger
3. Garlic

4. Cinnamon
5. Cumin
6. Paprika
7. Basil
8. Oregano
9. Rosemary

Condiments and Sauces:

1. Balsamic vinegar
2. Olive tapenade
3. Hummus
4. Soy sauce (low-sodium)
5. Mustard
6. Lemon juice

Frozen Section:

1. Frozen berries
2. Frozen vegetables (mixed varieties)

Beverages:

1. Herbal teas (ginger, mint, chamomile)
2. Water (for hydration)
3. Coconut water

Snacks:

1. Dark chocolate (in moderation)
2. Mixed nuts and seeds trail mix
3. Whole grain crackers

Sweeteners (Optional):

1. Honey
2. Maple syrup
3. Stevia

Miscellaneous:

1. Whole grain flour (for baking)
2. Dark chocolate chips (for baking)
3. Plant-based protein powder (optional)

CHAPTER THREE

Fruits Recipes

Mixed Berry Bliss Smoothie:

Meal Description: Start your day with a burst of flavor and energy by indulging in our Mixed Berry Bliss Smoothie. Packed with the goodness of antioxidant-rich mixed berries, the creaminess of banana, and the protein punch from Greek yogurt, this delightful smoothie perfectly balances taste and nutrition. Plus, it's a quick and easy way to kickstart your morning or enjoy a refreshing pick-me-up any time of the day.

Ingredients:

• 1 cup mixed berries (strawberries, blueberries, raspberries)

• One ripe banana

• 1/2 cup Greek yogurt

• 1/2 cup ice cubes (optional for a colder texture)

• 1/2 cup water or almond milk (adjust for desired consistency)

• One teaspoon of honey or maple syrup (optional for added sweetness)

Instructions:

1. Prepare Ingredients: Wash the mixed berries thoroughly and peel the banana.

2. Assemble Ingredients: In a blender, combine the mixed berries, peeled banana, Greek yogurt, and ice cubes.

3. Blend: Blend the ingredients on high speed until you achieve a smooth and creamy texture. Add water or almond milk gradually to reach your preferred

consistency.

4. Taste and Sweeten (Optional): Taste the smoothie and, if desired, add honey or maple syrup for a touch of sweetness. Blend again to incorporate.

5. Serve: Pour the smoothie into a glass and garnish with a few whole berries for an extra burst of freshness.

6. Enjoy: Sip and savor the delightful flavors of this Mixed Berry Bliss Smoothie as a wholesome breakfast or a healthy snack.

Nutrition Information (per serving):

• Calories: 200 calories

• Protein: 10g

• Carbohydrates: 40g

• Fat: 3g

• Fiber: 6g

MINTY FRESH FRUIT SALAD:

Meal Description: Quench your thirst and tantalize your taste buds with our Minty Fresh Fruit Salad. This hydrating and vibrant salad brings together the juiciness of watermelon, strawberries' sweetness, kiwi's tartness, and the refreshing hint of mint. It's the perfect ensemble for a light and revitalizing snack, ensuring you stay cool and energized throughout the day.

Ingredients:

• 2 cups cubed watermelon

• 1 cup sliced strawberries

• Two ripe kiwis, peeled and sliced

• Two tablespoons fresh mint leaves, finely chopped

• One tablespoon honey (optional for added sweetness)

Instructions:

1. Prepare Ingredients: Wash the watermelon, strawberries, and kiwis. Cut the watermelon into bite-sized cubes, slice the strawberries, and peel and slice the kiwis.

2. Combine Fruits: In a large mixing bowl, gently combine the cubed watermelon, sliced strawberries, and kiwi slices.

3. Add Mint: Sprinkle the finely chopped mint leaves over

the fruit mixture. The mint will add a refreshing element to the salad.

4. Optional Sweetening: If you prefer a slightly sweeter taste, drizzle honey over the fruit salad and gently toss to coat. Adjust the sweetness according to your preference.

5. Chill (Optional): For an extra refreshing experience, refrigerate the fruit salad for about 30 minutes before serving.

6. Serve Portion the Minty Fresh Fruit Salad in bowls or on a platter, ensuring an even distribution of fruits and mint.

7. Enjoy: Dive into this hydrating and invigorating fruit salad, savoring the delightful combination of flavors and textures.

Nutrition Information (per serving):

• Calories: 120 calories

• Protein: 2g

• Carbohydrates: 30g

• Fat: 1g

• Fiber: 5g

GRILLED PINEAPPLE SKEWERS:

Meal Description: Elevate your summer gatherings or satisfy your sweet cravings with these Grilled Pineapple Skewers. The natural sweetness of pineapple takes on a delightful caramelized flavor when grilled, creating a simple yet delicious treat. These skewers are perfect for a quick dessert, a flavorful side, or a refreshing snack on a warm day.

Ingredients:

• One medium pineapple, peeled, cored, and cut into chunks

• Wooden or metal skewers (if using wooden skewers, soak them in water for 30 minutes before grilling)

• Two tablespoons honey (optional for drizzling)

• Fresh mint leaves for garnish (optional)

Instructions:

1. Preheat the Grill: Preheat your grill to medium-high heat.

2. Prepare Pineapple: Cut the pineapple into bite-sized chunks, ensuring the core is removed.

3. Skewer the Pineapple: Thread the pineapple chunks onto the skewers. Leave a little space between each piece for even cooking.

4. Grill the Skewers: Place the skewers on the preheated grill. Grill for 2-3 minutes per side or until the pineapple develops grill marks and caramelizes slightly. Be attentive to avoid overcooking.

5. Optional Drizzle: If desired, drizzle honey over the grilled pineapple skewers while they are still hot. This adds an extra layer of sweetness and a glossy finish.

6. Garnish (Optional): Sprinkle fresh mint leaves over the skewers for a burst of color and added freshness.

7. Serve: Arrange the Grilled Pineapple Skewers on a platter and serve them immediately.

8. Enjoy: Dive into the delightful combination of smoky, caramelized, and sweet flavors with each bite of these Grilled Pineapple Skewers.

Nutrition Information (per serving):

• Calories: 80 calories

• Carbohydrates: 20g

• Fiber: 2g

• Sugars: 15g

• Fat: 0g

APPLE CINNAMON OATMEAL:

Meal Description: Warm, comforting, and bursting with fall flavors, our Apple Cinnamon Oatmeal is the perfect way to start your day. Combining the wholesome goodness of oats with the sweetness of apples and the warmth of cinnamon, this breakfast dish nourishes your body and fills your kitchen with a delightful aroma. It's a hearty and satisfying way to fuel your morning.

Ingredients:

• 1 cup old-fashioned rolled oats

• One medium-sized apple, peeled, cored, and diced

• One teaspoon ground cinnamon

• One tablespoon of honey or maple syrup (optional for added sweetness)

• 2 cups water or milk (dairy or plant-based)

• Pinch of salt

• Chopped nuts or raisins for topping (optional)

Instructions:

1. Cook Oats: Combine the oats and water or milk in a medium-sized saucepan. Add a pinch of salt. Bring to a boil, then reduce the heat to medium-low and simmer for 5-7

minutes or until the oats are tender, stirring occasionally.

2. Add Apples and Cinnamon: Stir in the diced apples and ground cinnamon. Continue to simmer for an additional 2-3 minutes, allowing the apples to soften and the flavors to meld.

3. Optional Sweetening: If desired, drizzle honey or maple syrup over the oatmeal for added sweetness. Stir well to combine.

4. Serve: Spoon the Apple Cinnamon Oatmeal into bowls.

5. Optional Toppings: Garnish with chopped nuts or raisins for added texture and flavor.

6. Enjoy: Dive into the heartwarming goodness of this Apple Cinnamon Oatmeal, savoring each spoonful of comforting oats and the natural sweetness of apples.

Nutrition Information (per serving):

• Calories: 250 calories

• Protein: 6g

• Carbohydrates: 50g

• Fiber: 7g

• Sugars: 20g

• Fat: 4g

CITRUS AVOCADO SALAD:

Meal Description: Elevate your salad game with our Citrus Avocado Salad. This vibrant and refreshing dish combines the citrusy goodness of oranges and grapefruit with the creamy texture of avocado. Packed with vitamin C and healthy fats, this salad not only delights your taste buds but also nourishes your body. It's a perfect side dish or a light, nutritious meal for any time of the day.

Ingredients:

• Two oranges, peeled and segmented

• One grapefruit, peeled and segmented

• One ripe avocado, peeled, pitted, and diced

• Mixed salad greens (e.g., arugula, spinach, or mixed greens)

• Two tablespoons extra-virgin olive oil

• One tablespoon of balsamic vinegar

• Salt and pepper to taste

• Optional: Fresh mint leaves for garnish

Instructions:

1. Prepare Citrus Segments: Peel and segment the oranges and grapefruit. Make sure to remove any seeds.

2. Dice Avocado: Peel, pit, and dice the ripe avocado.

3. Assemble Salad: In a large salad bowl, combine the citrus segments, diced avocado, and mixed salad greens.

4. Prepare Dressing: Whisk together the extra-virgin olive oil and balsamic vinegar in a small bowl. Season with salt and pepper to taste.

5. Dress the Salad: Drizzle the dressing over the salad and gently toss to coat the ingredients evenly.

6. Optional Garnish: For a burst of freshness, garnish the Citrus Avocado Salad with fresh mint leaves.

7. Serve: Portion the salad onto individual plates or a serving platter.

8. Enjoy Delight in this Citrus Avocado Salad's zesty and creamy flavors, savoring the combination of juicy citrus and buttery avocado.

Nutrition Information (per serving):

• Calories: 200 calories

• Protein: 3g

• Carbohydrates: 20g

• Fiber: 7g

• Sugars: 10g

• Fat: 14g

PEACH AND BLUEBERRY PARFAIT:

Meal Description: Indulge in the perfect harmony of sweetness and creaminess with our Peach and Blueberry Parfait. Layered with fresh, juicy peaches, plump blueberries, and rich Greek yogurt, this delightful parfait is a feast for the eyes and a treat for your taste buds. Enjoy it as a wholesome breakfast, a satisfying snack, or a guilt-free dessert.

Ingredients:

• Two ripe peaches, peeled and sliced

• 1 cup fresh blueberries

• 1 1/2 cups Greek yogurt (vanilla or plain)

• Two tablespoons honey or maple syrup (optional for drizzling)

• Granola for added crunch (optional)

Instructions:

1. Prepare Ingredients: Peel and slice the ripe peaches.

2. Layering the Parfait:

• In serving glasses or bowls, start by placing a layer of

Greek yogurt at the bottom.

• Add a layer of sliced peaches on top of the yogurt.

• Follow with a layer of fresh blueberries.

1. Repeat Layers: Repeat the layering process until the glass or bowl is filled, finishing with a dollop of Greek yogurt on top.

2. Optional Drizzle: If desired, drizzle honey or maple syrup over the top for added sweetness.

3. Optional Crunchy Topping: For an extra layer of texture, sprinkle granola over the parfait.

4. Repeat for Multiple Servings: Repeat the layering steps for additional servings.

5. Chill (Optional): For a refreshing touch, refrigerate the parfaits for about 15-30 minutes before serving.

6. Serve: Present these Peach and Blueberry Parfaits to dazzle your senses with their vibrant colors and delicious flavors.

7. Enjoy: Dive into the layers of goodness, relishing the combination of creamy yogurt, sweet peaches, and juicy blueberries.

Nutrition Information (per serving):

• Calories: 200 calories

• Protein: 15g

• Carbohydrates: 35g

• Fiber: 5g

• Sugars: 25g

• Fat: 4g

ORANGE GINGER TURMERIC SMOOTHIE:

Meal Description: Our Orange Ginger Turmeric Smoothie gives your immune system a powerful boost. Packed with the vitamin C goodness of oranges, the anti-inflammatory properties of ginger and turmeric, and the probiotics from yogurt, this smoothie is a tasty and nutritious way to kickstart your day or provide a refreshing pick-me-up. Let the vibrant colors and zesty flavors invigorate your senses.

Ingredients:

• Two oranges, peeled and segmented

• One tablespoon of fresh ginger, peeled and grated

• 1/2 teaspoon ground turmeric

• 1 cup plain or Greek yogurt

• One tablespoon of honey or maple syrup (optional for added sweetness)

• 1/2 cup ice cubes (optional for a colder texture)

Instructions:

1. Prepare Ingredients: Peel and segment the oranges. Peel and grate the fresh ginger.

2. Blend: In a blender, combine the orange segments, grated ginger, ground turmeric, yogurt, and ice cubes (if using).

3. Optional Sweetening: If desired, add honey or maple syrup for sweetness.

4. Blend Until Smooth: Blend all the ingredients until you achieve a smooth and creamy consistency.

5. Taste and Adjust: Taste the smoothie and adjust the sweetness or thickness by adding more honey, yogurt, or ice cubes if necessary. Blend again as needed.

6. Serve: Pour the Orange Ginger Turmeric Smoothie into a glass.

7. Optional Garnish: Garnish with a slice of orange or a sprinkle of turmeric for an extra visual appeal.

8. Enjoy: Sip and savor the refreshing flavors of this immune-boosting smoothie, knowing that you're nourishing your body with powerful antioxidants and nutrients.

Nutrition Information (per serving):

• Calories: 150 calories

• Protein: 8g

• Carbohydrates: 30g

• Fiber: 4g

• Sugars: 20g

• Fat: 2g

CHAPTER FOUR

Vegetables recipes

Roasted Vegetable Quinoa Bowl:

Meal Description: Elevate your mealtime with our Roasted Vegetable Quinoa Bowl—a colorful and nutrient-packed dish that combines the earthy flavors of roasted zucchini, vibrant bell peppers, and burst-in-your-mouth cherry tomatoes over a bed of protein-rich quinoa. This wholesome bowl satisfies your taste buds and provides a balanced and nourishing experience.

Ingredients:

For Roasted Vegetables:

• One medium zucchini, sliced

• One red bell pepper, sliced

• One yellow bell pepper, sliced

• 1 cup cherry tomatoes, halved

• Two tablespoons olive oil

• One teaspoon of dried thyme

• Salt and pepper to taste

For Quinoa:

• 1 cup quinoa, rinsed

• 2 cups water or vegetable broth

• Salt to taste

Optional Toppings:

• Crumbled feta cheese

• Fresh basil or parsley, chopped

• Balsamic glaze for drizzling

Instructions:

1. Preheat the Oven: Preheat your oven to 400°F (200°C).

2. Prepare Vegetables: In a large mixing bowl, toss the sliced zucchini, bell peppers, and halved cherry tomatoes with olive oil, dried thyme, salt, and pepper until well coated.

3. Roast Vegetables: Spread the seasoned vegetables evenly on a baking sheet lined with parchment paper. Roast in the preheated oven for 20-25 minutes or until the vegetables are tender and slightly caramelized, stirring halfway through.

4. Prepare Quinoa: While the vegetables are roasting, rinse the quinoa under cold water. In a saucepan, combine the quinoa with water or vegetable broth and a pinch of salt. Bring to a boil, then reduce heat, cover, and simmer for 15-20 minutes or until the quinoa is cooked and the liquid is absorbed. Fluff the quinoa with a fork.

5. Assemble Bowls: Divide the cooked quinoa among serving bowls. Top with the roasted vegetables.

6. Optional Toppings: Sprinkle crumbled feta cheese and fresh basil or parsley over the bowls. Drizzle with balsamic glaze for added flavor.

7. Serve: Present these vibrant Roasted Vegetable Quinoa Bowls and enjoy a wholesome, flavorful meal.

8. Enjoy: Savor the delicious combination of roasted vegetables and fluffy quinoa, and customize each bite with your favorite toppings.

Nutrition Information (per serving, without optional toppings):

• Calories: 350 calories

- Protein: 10g
- Carbohydrates: 60g
- Fiber: 8g
- Sugars: 6g
- Fat: 10g

STIR-FRIED BROCCOLI AND TOFU:

Meal Description: Savor the flavors of a quick and healthy meal with our Stir-Fried Broccoli and Tofu. This dish combines the vibrant broccoli crunch, protein-packed goodness of Tofu, and the aromatic blend of garlic and ginger. This simple stir-fry satisfies your taste buds and provides a nutritious and satisfying option for a speedy lunch or dinner.

Ingredients:

For Stir-Fry:

- One block of firm Tofu pressed and cubed

- 3 cups broccoli florets

- Two tablespoons of vegetable oil

- Three cloves garlic, minced

- One tablespoon of fresh ginger, grated

- Two tablespoons soy sauce (or tamari for a gluten-free option)

- One tablespoon of sesame oil

- One tablespoon of rice vinegar

- One teaspoon sriracha sauce (optional, for heat)

- Salt and pepper to taste

For Serving:

- Cooked brown rice or quinoa

- Sesame seeds for garnish

- Chopped green onions for garnish

Instructions:

1. Prepare Tofu: Press the Tofu to remove excess water, then cut it into bite-sized cubes.

2. Stir-Fry Tofu: Heat vegetable oil in a large wok or skillet over medium-high heat. Add tofu cubes and cook until they are golden brown on all sides. Remove Tofu from the pan and set aside.

3. Stir-Fry Vegetables: Add a bit more oil, if needed, in the same pan. Add minced garlic and grated ginger, sautéing for about 30 seconds until fragrant. Add broccoli florets and stir-fry for 3-5 minutes until they are tender-crisp.

4. Combine Tofu and Broccoli: Return the cooked Tofu to the pan with the broccoli.

5. Prepare Sauce: In a small bowl, whisk together soy sauce, sesame oil, rice vinegar, and sriracha sauce (if using).

6. Add Sauce: Pour the sauce over the Tofu and broccoli. Toss everything together until well coated. Season with salt and pepper to taste.

7. Serve: Serve the stir-fried broccoli and Tofu over cooked brown rice or quinoa.

8. Garnish: Sprinkle sesame seeds and chopped green onions over the top for added flavor and texture.

9. Enjoy: Dive into a plate of this Stir-Fried Broccoli and Tofu, savoring the delightful combination of textures and savory flavors.

Nutrition Information (per serving, without rice/quinoa):

• Calories: 250 calories

• Protein: 20g

• Carbohydrates: 15g

• Fiber: 5g

• Sugars: 3g

• Fat: 15g

BUTTERNUT SQUASH SOUP:

Meal Description: Indulge in our Butternut Squash Soup's rich, velvety goodness. This comforting soup is made from roasted butternut squash blended with flavorful vegetable broth and is a warm embrace on chilly days. The squash's natural sweetness combined with aromatic spices creates a delightful harmony of flavors, making it a perfect appetizer or a light, nourishing meal.

Ingredients:

• One medium-sized butternut squash, peeled, seeded, and diced

• One onion, chopped

• Two cloves garlic, minced

• Two tablespoons olive oil

• 4 cups vegetable broth

• One teaspoon ground cinnamon

• 1/2 teaspoon ground nutmeg

• Salt and pepper to taste

• 1 cup unsweetened coconut milk (optional for creaminess)

• Fresh parsley or chives for garnish (optional)

Instructions:

1. Preheat Oven: Preheat your oven to 400°F (200°C).

2. Roast Butternut Squash: In a large bowl, toss the diced butternut squash with olive oil, salt, and pepper. Spread the squash on a baking sheet and roast in the preheated oven for 25-30 minutes or until tender and slightly caramelized.

3. Sauté Onion and Garlic: Heat a bit of olive oil over medium heat in a large pot. Add chopped onions and sauté until translucent. Add minced garlic and sauté for an additional 1-2 minutes.

4. Add Roasted Squash: Transfer the roasted butternut squash to the pot with onions and garlic.

5. Spice it Up: Sprinkle ground cinnamon and nutmeg over the squash. Stir to coat the ingredients with the spices.

6. Add Vegetable Broth: Pour in the vegetable broth. Bring the mixture to a boil, then reduce the heat and let it simmer for about 10-15 minutes to allow the flavors to meld.

7. Blend: Use an immersion blender or transfer the soup to a blender (in batches if necessary) and blend until smooth.

8. Adjust Consistency: Add coconut milk to achieve a creamier consistency if desired. Adjust salt and pepper to taste.

9. Serve: Ladle the Butternut Squash Soup into bowls.

10. Garnish (Optional): Garnish with fresh parsley or chives for a pop of color and added freshness.

11. Enjoy: Savor this Butternut Squash Soup's comforting warmth and delicious flavors.

Nutrition Information (per serving):

• Calories: 150 calories

- Protein: 2g
- Carbohydrates: 25g
- Fiber: 5g
- Sugars: 5g
- Fat: 7g

CUCUMBER AND TOMATO SALAD:

Meal Description: Experience summer's crisp and refreshing flavors with our Cucumber and Tomato Salad. This simple yet vibrant side dish combines the juiciness of cherry tomatoes, the cool crunch of cucumber, and the fragrant notes of fresh herbs, all tossed in a light olive oil dressing. Enjoy this salad as a refreshing accompaniment to your favorite meals or as a standalone snack on warm days.

Ingredients:

- Two large cucumbers, sliced

- 1 pint cherry tomatoes, halved

- Two tablespoons extra-virgin olive oil

- One tablespoon of balsamic vinegar

- One tablespoon of fresh lemon juice

- One teaspoon of Dijon mustard

- One clove garlic, minced (optional)

- Salt and pepper to taste

- Fresh basil or parsley, chopped, for garnish

- Feta cheese, crumbled (optional)

Instructions:

1. Prepare Vegetables: Slice the cucumbers and halve the cherry tomatoes.

2. Make Dressing: In a small bowl, whisk together the olive oil, balsamic vinegar, fresh lemon juice, Dijon mustard, minced garlic (if using), salt, and pepper.

3. Combine Vegetables: In a large salad bowl, combine the sliced cucumbers and halved cherry tomatoes.

4. Toss with Dressing: Pour the dressing over the vegetables. Toss gently to coat the vegetables evenly with the dressing.

5. Chill (Optional): For enhanced flavor, refrigerate the salad for about 15-30 minutes before serving.

6. Garnish: Just before serving, sprinkle chopped fresh basil or parsley over the salad. If desired, add crumbled feta cheese for an extra burst of flavor.

7. Serve: Spoon the Cucumber and Tomato Salad onto a serving platter or individual plates.

8. Enjoy Delight in this summer-inspired salad's crisp, refreshing taste as a side or a standalone snack.

Nutrition Information (per serving, without optional toppings):

• Calories: 80 calories

• Protein: 2g

• Carbohydrates: 8g

• Fiber: 2g

• Sugars: 4g

• Fat: 5g

SPINACH AND FETA STUFFED BELL PEPPERS:

Meal Description: Elevate your dinner with our Spinach and Feta Stuffed Bell Peppers—a delightful combination of vibrant bell peppers filled with a flavorful mixture of spinach, feta, and quinoa. This nutritious and satisfying dish looks impressive and delivers a burst of Mediterranean-inspired flavors. Perfect for a wholesome weeknight dinner or as a crowd-pleasing centerpiece for a special occasion.

Ingredients:

• Four large bell peppers (any color)

• 1 cup cooked quinoa

• 2 cups fresh spinach, chopped

• 1 cup crumbled feta cheese

• 1/2 cup cherry tomatoes, diced

• Two cloves garlic, minced

• One tablespoon olive oil

• One teaspoon dried oregano

• Salt and pepper to taste

• Fresh basil or parsley for garnish

Instructions:

1. Preheat the Oven: Preheat your oven to 375°F (190°C).

2. Prepare Bell Peppers: Cut the tops off the bell peppers and remove seeds and membranes. If needed, slice a small portion off the bottom of each pepper to make them stand upright.

3. Sauté Spinach and Garlic: Heat olive oil over medium heat in a skillet. Add minced garlic and sauté until fragrant. Add chopped spinach and cook until wilted. Season with salt and pepper.

4. Prepare Filling: In a mixing bowl, combine the cooked quinoa, sautéed spinach and garlic, crumbled feta cheese, diced cherry tomatoes, and dried oregano. Mix well.

5. Stuff Peppers: Spoon the quinoa mixture into each bell pepper, pressing it down gently. Continue until each pepper is filled.

6. Bake: Place the stuffed peppers in a baking dish. Bake in the preheated oven for 25-30 minutes or until the peppers are tender.

7. Garnish: Remove the stuffed peppers from the oven and garnish with fresh basil or parsley.

8. Serve: Arrange the Spinach and Feta Stuffed Bell Peppers on a serving platter.

9. Enjoy Delight in the savory goodness of these stuffed peppers, relishing the blend of spinach, feta, and quinoa.

Nutrition Information (per stuffed pepper):

• Calories: 250 calories

• Protein: 12g

- Carbohydrates: 30g
- Fiber: 5g
- Sugars: 5g
- Fat: 10g

ZUCCHINI NOODLES WITH PESTO:

Meal Description: Indulge in a light and flavorful dish with our Zucchini Noodles with Pesto—a delightful, low-carb alternative to traditional pasta. Spiralized zucchini takes center stage, tossed in a vibrant homemade pesto that's bursting with the freshness of basil, the richness of pine nuts, and the zing of garlic. This quick and healthy recipe is perfect for a satisfying weeknight dinner.

Ingredients:

For Zucchini Noodles:

• Four medium-sized zucchinis, spiralized

• Salt for sprinkling

For Pesto:

• 2 cups fresh basil leaves, packed

• 1/2 cup grated Parmesan cheese

• 1/2 cup pine nuts, toasted

• Three cloves garlic

• 1/2 cup extra-virgin olive oil

• Salt and pepper to taste

• Juice of half a lemon (optional)

Instructions:

1. Spiralize Zucchini: Use a spiralizer to create zucchini noodles. Sprinkle the noodles with salt and let them sit in a colander for about 15-20 minutes to release excess moisture. Pat them dry with a paper towel.

2. Toast Pine Nuts: In a dry skillet over medium heat, toast the pine nuts until golden brown, stirring frequently to prevent burning. Set aside to cool.

3. Prepare Pesto: In a food processor, combine fresh basil, grated Parmesan cheese, toasted pine nuts, and garlic. Pulse until finely chopped.

4. Add Olive Oil: With the food processor running, gradually add the olive oil in a steady stream. Continue processing until the pesto reaches your desired consistency.

5. Season and Adjust: Season the pesto with salt and pepper. If desired, add lemon juice for a hint of brightness. Adjust the seasoning to taste.

6. Toss Zucchini Noodles: In a large bowl, toss the spiralized zucchini noodles with the homemade pesto until well-coated.

7. Serve: Portion the Zucchini Noodles with Pesto onto plates.

8. Optional Garnish: Garnish with additional Parmesan cheese and a sprinkle of toasted pine nuts.

9. Enjoy: Relish the freshness and vibrant flavors of this low-carb pasta alternative.

Nutrition Information (per serving):

· Calories: 250 calories

- Protein: 8g
- Carbohydrates: 10g
- Fiber: 4g
- Sugars: 4g
- Fat: 20g

EGGPLANT AND TOMATO STACK:

Meal Description: Experience the elegance of simplicity with our Eggplant and Tomato Stack—a light and flavorful dish that showcases the natural goodness of roasted eggplant, ripe tomatoes, and fragrant basil. Layers of these fresh ingredients come together to create a visually stunning and delicious stack. Perfect as a light lunch, appetizer, or a side dish for a Mediterranean-inspired feast.

Ingredients:

• One large eggplant, thinly sliced

• Two large tomatoes, thinly sliced

• Fresh basil leaves

• Olive oil for brushing

• Balsamic glaze for drizzling (optional)

• Salt and pepper to taste

Instructions:

1. Preheat the Oven: Preheat your oven to 400°F (200°C).

2. Prepare Eggplant: Slice the eggplant into thin rounds. Place the slices on a paper towel, sprinkle with salt, and let them sit for about 15 minutes to release excess moisture. Pat the eggplant slices dry with another paper towel.

3. Roast Eggplant: Brush the eggplant slices with olive oil and place them on a baking sheet. Roast in the preheated oven for 15-20 minutes or until the slices are tender and golden brown, flipping halfway through.

4. Layer Stacks: Assemble the stacks by layering a slice of roasted eggplant, a slice of tomato, and a basil leaf. Repeat the layering until you reach the desired height, finishing with a basil leaf on top.

5. Season: Sprinkle salt and pepper over the top of each stack to taste.

6. Optional Drizzle: Drizzle balsamic glaze over the stacks for an extra burst of flavor.

7. Serve: Carefully transfer the Eggplant and Tomato Stacks to serving plates.

8. Enjoy: Savor the freshness and harmonious flavors of this elegant dish. Each bite brings together the creamy texture of eggplant, the juiciness of tomatoes, and the aromatic essence of basil.

Note: You can serve these stacks warm or at room temperature.

Nutrition Information (per serving):

• Calories: 80 calories

• Protein: 2g

• Carbohydrates: 10g

• Fiber: 4g

• Sugars: 5g

• Fat: 4g

CHAPTER FIVE

Whole Grains Recipes

Quinoa Salad with Chickpeas:

Meal Description: Enjoy a nutritious and satisfying meal with our Quinoa Salad with Chickpeas—a refreshing and protein-packed dish that combines fluffy quinoa, hearty chickpeas, crisp cucumber, and a zesty lemon vinaigrette. This vibrant salad is quick to prepare and versatile enough to serve as a light lunch, a side dish, or a wholesome dinner option.

Ingredients:

For the Salad:

- 1 cup quinoa, cooked and cooled

- One can (15 oz) chickpeas, drained and rinsed

- One cucumber, diced

- 1/2 red onion, finely chopped

- 1/4 cup fresh parsley, chopped

- Salt and pepper to taste

For the Lemon Vinaigrette:

- 1/4 cup extra-virgin olive oil

- Zest and juice of 1 lemon

- One teaspoon of Dijon mustard

- One clove of garlic, minced

- Salt and pepper to taste

Instructions:

1. Prepare Quinoa: Cook quinoa according to package instructions. Once cooked, let it cool to room temperature.

2. Make Lemon Vinaigrette: In a small bowl, whisk together olive oil, lemon zest, lemon juice, Dijon mustard, minced garlic, salt, and pepper to create the lemon vinaigrette.

3. Assemble Salad: In a large mixing bowl, combine the cooked and cooled quinoa, chickpeas, diced cucumber, chopped red onion, and fresh parsley.

4. Drizzle with Vinaigrette: Pour the lemon vinaigrette over the salad ingredients. Toss the salad gently to coat everything evenly with the vinaigrette.

5. Season: Season the salad with additional salt and pepper to taste.

6. Chill (Optional): For enhanced flavors, refrigerate the salad for about 15-30 minutes before serving.

7. Serve: Portion the Quinoa Salad with Chickpeas onto individual plates or a serving platter.

8. Enjoy Delight in the combination of textures and flavors in each bite of this wholesome and satisfying quinoa salad.

Nutrition Information (per serving):

• Calories: 300 calories

• Protein: 10g

• Carbohydrates: 40g

• Fiber: 7g

• Sugars: 3g

• Fat: 14g

BROWN RICE AND VEGETABLE STIR-FRY:

Meal Description: Embark on a culinary journey with our Brown Rice and Vegetable Stir-Fry—a wholesome and flavorful dish that brings together nutty brown rice, a colorful assortment of vegetables, and your choice of protein, whether it's tofu or shrimp. This stir-fry is a delicious and nutritious way to enjoy a well-balanced meal's vibrant textures and tastes.

Ingredients:

For Stir-Fry:

• 2 cups cooked brown rice, cooled

• 1 cup tofu, cubed (or shrimp, peeled and deveined)

• 2 cups mixed vegetables (e.g., broccoli, bell peppers, snap peas, carrots), chopped

• Two tablespoons of vegetable oil

• Three cloves garlic, minced

• One tablespoon of fresh ginger, grated

• Soy sauce or tamari for seasoning

• Salt and pepper to taste

- Green onions, chopped, for garnish (optional)

- Sesame seeds for garnish (optional)

For Sauce:

- Three tablespoons soy sauce or tamari

- One tablespoon of hoisin sauce

- One tablespoon of rice vinegar

- One teaspoon of sesame oil

- One teaspoon of honey or maple syrup (optional for sweetness)

Instructions:

1. Prepare Sauce: In a small bowl, whisk together soy sauce, hoisin sauce, rice vinegar, sesame oil, and honey (if using) to create the sauce. Set aside.

2. Cook Protein: Heat 1 tablespoon of vegetable oil over medium-high heat in a large skillet or wok. Add cubed tofu or shrimp, cooking until tofu is golden brown or shrimp are cooked through. Remove from the pan and set aside.

3. Stir-Fry Vegetables: Add another tablespoon of vegetable oil in the same pan. Add minced garlic and grated ginger, sautéing for about 30 seconds until fragrant. Add the chopped vegetables and stir-fry until they are tender-crisp.

4. Combine Rice: Add the cooked and cooled brown rice to the pan, stirring to combine with the vegetables.

5. Add Protein: Return the cooked tofu or shrimp to the pan, mixing it with the rice and vegetables.

6. Pour Sauce: Pour the prepared sauce over the rice and vegetable mixture. Toss everything together until well coated.

7. Season: Season the stir-fry with soy sauce or tamari, salt, and pepper to taste. Adjust the seasoning as needed.

8. Garnish (Optional): Garnish with chopped green onions and sesame seeds for added flavor and visual appeal.

9. Serve: Portion the Brown Rice and Vegetable Stir-Fry onto plates or into bowls.

10. Enjoy: Savor the delightful combination of textures and flavors in each forkful of this wholesome stir-fry.

Nutrition Information (per serving):

• Calories: 350 calories

• Protein: 15g

• Carbohydrates: 55g

• Fiber: 8g

• Sugars: 5g

• Fat: 12g

WHOLE GRAIN PASTA WITH PESTO AND CHERRY TOMATOES:

Meal Description: Delight in the wholesome goodness of our Whole Grain Pasta with Pesto and Cherry Tomatoes—a flavorful and nutritious dish that combines the heartiness of whole grain pasta, the vibrant freshness of cherry tomatoes, and the rich zing of homemade pesto. This quick and easy recipe is a celebration of simple ingredients that come together to create a satisfying and delicious meal.

Ingredients:

• 8 oz (about 225g) whole grain pasta (such as whole wheat or multigrain)

• 1 pint cherry tomatoes, halved

• Fresh basil leaves for garnish

For Pesto:

• 2 cups fresh basil leaves, packed

• 1/2 cup grated Parmesan cheese

• 1/2 cup pine nuts, toasted

• Two cloves garlic

• 1/2 cup extra-virgin olive oil

• Salt and pepper to taste

• Juice of half a lemon (optional)

Instructions:

1. Cook Pasta: Cook the whole grain pasta according to package instructions until al dente. Drain and set aside.

2. Make Pesto: In a food processor, combine fresh basil, grated Parmesan cheese, toasted pine nuts, and garlic. Pulse until finely chopped.

3. Add Olive Oil: With the food processor running, gradually add the olive oil in a steady stream. Continue processing until the pesto reaches your desired consistency.

4. Season and Adjust: Season the pesto with salt and pepper. If desired, add lemon juice for a hint of brightness. Adjust the seasoning to taste.

5. Toss Pasta and Tomatoes: In a large mixing bowl, toss the cooked whole-grain pasta with the homemade pesto until the pasta is well coated. Add the halved cherry tomatoes and gently toss again.

6. Optional Garnish: Garnish with fresh basil leaves for an extra burst of flavor.

7. Serve: Portion the Whole Grain Pasta with Pesto and Cherry Tomatoes onto plates or into bowls.

8. Enjoy: Savor each forkful of this wholesome pasta dish, appreciating the harmony of textures and flavors.

Nutrition Information (per serving):

- Calories: 350 calories
- Protein: 10g
- Carbohydrates: 40g
- Fiber: 8g
- Sugars: 5g
- Fat: 20g

BARLEY AND MUSHROOM RISOTTO:

Meal Description: Indulge in the comforting richness of our Barley and Mushroom Risotto—a hearty twist on the classic using nutty barley, earthy mushrooms, and the savory depth of Parmesan cheese. This wholesome and satisfying dish is a celebration of flavors and textures that will warm your soul and become a favorite in your culinary repertoire.

Ingredients:

• 1 cup pearl barley

• 4 cups vegetable or chicken broth

• Two tablespoons olive oil

• One onion, finely chopped

• Two cloves garlic, minced

• 8 oz (about 225g) mushrooms (such as cremini or button), sliced

• 1/2 cup dry white wine (optional)

• 1/2 cup grated Parmesan cheese

• Salt and pepper to taste

• Fresh parsley, chopped, for garnish

Instructions:

1. Prepare Broth: Heat the vegetable or chicken broth in a saucepan until it simmers. Keep it warm over low heat.

2. Sauté Onion and Garlic: Heat olive oil over medium heat in a large skillet or wide saucepan. Add finely chopped onion and sauté until translucent. Add minced garlic and cook for an additional 1-2 minutes.

3. Add Barley: Stir in the pearl barley, ensuring it is well coated with the onion and garlic mixture.

4. Deglaze with Wine (Optional): Pour in the white wine (if using) and stir, allowing it to deglaze the pan. Cook until most of the wine has evaporated.

5. Begin Adding Broth: Start adding the warm broth, one ladleful at a time, stirring frequently. Allow the barley to absorb the broth before adding the next ladleful. Continue this process until the barley is cooked, which may take about 30-40 minutes. The barley should be tender with a slight chewiness.

6. Sauté Mushrooms: In a separate pan, sauté the sliced mushrooms in a bit of olive oil until they are golden brown and have released their moisture.

7. Combine Mushrooms: Mix the sautéed mushrooms with the barley risotto.

8. Finish and Season: Stir in the grated Parmesan cheese once the barley is cooked to your liking. Season the risotto with salt and pepper to taste.

9. Garnish: Garnish the Barley and Mushroom Risotto with chopped fresh parsley.

10. Serve: Portion the risotto onto plates or into bowls.

11. Enjoy: Savor the heartiness and depth of flavors in each spoonful of this satisfying Barley and Mushroom Risotto.

Note: Adjust the consistency of the risotto by adding more broth or water if needed.

Nutrition Information (per serving):

• Calories: 350 calories

• Protein: 10g

• Carbohydrates: 55g

• Fiber: 8g

• Sugars: 3g

• Fat: 10g

FARRO AND VEGETABLE SOUP:

Meal Description: Embrace the warmth and nourishment of our Farro and Vegetable Soup—a hearty and wholesome blend of nutty farro, vibrant carrots, crisp celery, and tender spinach. This comforting soup is packed with nutritious ingredients and offers a symphony of flavors that will satisfy your taste buds and keep you cozy on chilly days.

Ingredients:

- 1 cup farro, rinsed

- One tablespoon olive oil

- One onion, chopped

- Two carrots diced

- Two celery stalks, diced

- Three cloves garlic, minced

- 8 cups vegetable broth

- One can (15 oz) diced tomatoes, undrained

- One teaspoon of dried thyme

- One teaspoon of dried rosemary

- Salt and pepper to taste

• 2 cups fresh spinach, chopped

• Fresh parsley, chopped, for garnish

• Grated Parmesan cheese for serving (optional)

Instructions:

1. Prepare Farro: Rinse the Farro under cold water.

2. Sauté Vegetables: Heat olive oil over medium heat in a large pot. Add chopped onion, diced carrots, and diced celery. Sauté until the vegetables are softened, about 5-7 minutes.

3. Add Garlic: Add minced garlic to the pot and sauté for an additional 1-2 minutes until fragrant.

4. Combine Broth: Pour in the vegetable broth, dice the tomatoes (with their juices), and rinse the farro. Stir in dried thyme and dried rosemary. Bring the mixture to a boil.

5. Simmer Soup: Reduce the heat to low, cover the pot, and let the soup simmer for about 20-25 minutes or until the farro is tender.

6. Season: Season the soup with salt and pepper to taste. Adjust the seasoning as needed.

7. Add Spinach: Stir in the chopped fresh spinach and let it wilt into the soup.

8. Garnish: Garnish the Farro and Vegetable Soup with chopped fresh parsley.

9. Serve: Ladle the soup into bowls.

10. Optional Topping: Optionally, serve the soup with a sprinkle of grated Parmesan cheese on top.

11. Enjoy the nourishing warmth and delightful

combination of flavors in each spoonful of this Farro and Vegetable Soup.

Note: You can customize the soup by adding other vegetables like zucchini, bell peppers, or kale.

Nutrition Information (per serving):

• Calories: 250 calories

• Protein: 8g

• Carbohydrates: 50g

• Fiber: 8g

• Sugars: 5g

• Fat: 4g

WILD RICE PILAF WITH CRANBERRIES:

Meal Description: Experience the delightful blend of earthy flavors and vibrant colors with our Wild Rice Pilaf with Cranberries—a festive and flavorful dish that brings together the nuttiness of wild rice, the tartness of cranberries, the crunch of almonds, and a hint of citrusy zest. This dish is perfect for holiday gatherings or as a unique side dish that adds a burst of flavor and elegance to your table.

Ingredients:

• 1 cup wild rice

• 2 cups vegetable or chicken broth

• 1/2 cup dried cranberries

• 1/2 cup slivered almonds, toasted

• Zest one orange

• Two tablespoons olive oil

• One small onion, finely chopped

• Two cloves garlic, minced

• Salt and pepper to taste

• Fresh parsley, chopped, for garnish

Instructions:

1. Rinse and Cook Wild Rice: Rinse the wild rice under cold water. In a saucepan, combine the wild rice and broth. Bring to a boil, then reduce the heat, cover, and simmer for about 45-60 minutes or until the rice is tender and has absorbed the liquid.

2. Prepare Cranberries: In a small bowl, soak the dried cranberries in warm water for about 10 minutes to plump them up. Drain and set aside.

3. Toast Almonds: In a dry skillet over medium heat, toast the slivered almonds until they are golden brown, stirring frequently. Remove from the skillet and set aside.

4. Sauté Onion and Garlic: Heat olive oil over medium heat in the same skillet. Add finely chopped onion and sauté until translucent. Add minced garlic and cook for an additional 1-2 minutes.

5. Combine Ingredients: Add the cooked wild rice, plumped cranberries, toasted almonds, and orange zest to the skillet. Stir everything together until well combined.

6. Season: Season the pilaf with salt and pepper to taste. Adjust the seasoning as needed.

7. Garnish: Garnish the Wild Rice Pilaf with Cranberries with chopped fresh parsley.

8. Serve: Spoon the pilaf onto a serving platter or individual plates.

9. Enjoy: Savor the delightful combination of textures and flavors in each forkful of this festive Wild Rice Pilaf with Cranberries.

Note: Feel free to add fresh herbs like thyme or rosemary for an extra layer of flavor.

Nutrition Information (per serving):

- Calories: 250 calories
- Protein: 8g
- Carbohydrates: 40g
- Fiber: 5g
- Sugars: 8g
- Fat: 8g

BUCKWHEAT PANCAKES WITH BERRIES:

Meal Description: Start your morning with a wholesome and flavorful breakfast by indulging in our Buckwheat Pancakes with Berries—a stack of hearty pancakes made with nutty buckwheat flour and topped with a vibrant assortment of fresh berries. These pancakes offer a delightful combination of textures and flavors and provide a nutritious and satisfying start to your day.

Ingredients:

For Buckwheat Pancakes:

• 1 cup buckwheat flour

• One tablespoon sugar

• One teaspoon of baking powder

• 1/2 teaspoon baking soda

• 1/4 teaspoon salt

• 1 cup buttermilk

• One large egg

• Two tablespoons melted butter (or oil)

• Cooking spray or additional butter for greasing the pan

For Topping:

• Mixed berries (strawberries, blueberries, raspberries)

• Maple syrup

• Greek yogurt (optional)

Instructions:

1. Prepare Dry Ingredients: In a mixing bowl, whisk together buckwheat flour, sugar, baking powder, baking soda, and salt.

2. Mix Wet Ingredients: In a separate bowl, whisk together buttermilk, egg, and melted butter (or oil).

3. Combine Wet and Dry Ingredients: Pour the wet ingredients into the dry ingredients and gently mix until just combined. Do not overmix; a few lumps are okay.

4. Preheat Pan: Heat a non-stick skillet or griddle over medium heat. If needed, lightly grease the surface with cooking spray or a small amount of butter.

5. Cook Pancakes: Pour 1/4 cup portions of batter onto the hot skillet to form pancakes. Cook until bubbles form on the surface, then flip and cook the other side until golden brown.

6. Repeat the process until all the batter is used, adjusting the heat if necessary.

7. Assemble Pancake Stack: Stack the cooked buckwheat pancakes on a plate.

8. Top with Berries: Generously top the pancake stack with a mixture of fresh berries.

9. Drizzle with Syrup: Drizzle maple syrup over the pancakes and berries.

10. Optional Yogurt Topping: Add a dollop of Greek yogurt on top for an extra touch.

11. Serve: Serve the Buckwheat Pancakes with Berries while warm.

12. Enjoy: Enjoy the delightful combination of nutty buckwheat pancakes and the sweetness of fresh berries.

Note: You can customize the toppings with additional nuts, seeds, or a dusting of powdered sugar.

Nutrition Information (per serving):

• Calories: 250 calories

• Protein: 7g

• Carbohydrates: 40g

• Fiber: 5g

• Sugars: 10g

• Fat: 8g

CHAPTER SIX

Fatty Fish recipes

Grilled Salmon with Lemon-Dill Sauce:

Meal Description: Elevate your dinner with the delightful combination of succulent grilled salmon and a zesty Lemon-Dill Sauce. This dish not only brings out the natural flavors of the salmon but also adds a refreshing and herby touch with the yogurt-based sauce. Enjoy a healthy and delicious meal that's perfect for any occasion.

Ingredients:

For Grilled Salmon:

• Four salmon fillets

• Two tablespoons olive oil

• One teaspoon of lemon zest

• One tablespoon of lemon juice

• Salt and pepper to taste

• Fresh dill for garnish

For Lemon-Dill Sauce:

• 1/2 cup Greek yogurt

• One tablespoon of fresh dill, finely chopped

• One tablespoon of lemon juice

• One teaspoon of lemon zest

• Salt and pepper to taste

Instructions:

1. Preheat Grill: Preheat your grill to medium-high heat.

2. Prepare Salmon Marinade: In a small bowl, mix together olive oil, lemon zest, lemon juice, salt, and pepper.

3. Marinate Salmon: Place the salmon fillets on a plate or in a shallow dish. Brush the marinade over both sides of each fillet, ensuring they are well coated. Let them marinate for at least 15-30 minutes.

4. Make Lemon-Dill Sauce: In a separate bowl, combine Greek yogurt, chopped fresh dill, lemon juice, lemon zest, salt, and pepper. Stir well to create the Lemon-Dill Sauce. Adjust the seasoning to taste.

5. Grill Salmon: Place the marinated salmon fillets on the preheated grill. Grill for about 4-6 minutes per side or until the salmon is cooked to your preferred level of doneness. The internal temperature should reach 145°F (63°C).

6. Serve: Transfer the grilled salmon fillets to a serving platter.

7. Top with Lemon-Dill Sauce: Spoon the Lemon-Dill Sauce over each grilled salmon fillet.

8. Garnish: Garnish with additional fresh dill for a burst of color and flavor.

9. Serve Warm: Serve the Grilled Salmon with Lemon-Dill Sauce while warm.

10. Enjoy: Relish the smoky grilled salmon's perfect harmony and the Lemon-Dill Sauce's zesty freshness.

Note: You can serve the grilled salmon with your choice of sides, such as roasted vegetables, quinoa, or a light salad.

Nutrition Information (per serving):

• Calories: 300 calories

• Protein: 30g

• Carbohydrates: 3g

• Sugars: 1g

- Fat: 20g

BAKED COD WITH HERBS:

Meal Description: Enjoy a light and flavorful dinner with our Baked Cod with Herbs—a simple and healthy dish that features flaky cod fillets infused with the aromatic blend of herbs and garlic. Baking the cod in olive oil ensures a moist and tender result, making this recipe both delicious and easy to prepare.

Ingredients:

• Four cod fillets

• Two tablespoons olive oil

• Two cloves garlic, minced

• One teaspoon of dried thyme

• One teaspoon of dried rosemary

• One teaspoon dried oregano

• Salt and pepper to taste

• Lemon wedges for serving

• Fresh parsley, chopped, for garnish

Instructions:

1. Preheat Oven: Preheat your oven to 375°F (190°C).

2. Prepare Baking Dish: Grease a baking dish with a bit of

olive oil or use parchment paper to prevent sticking.

3. Season Cod Fillets: Pat the cod fillets dry with a paper towel. Place them in the prepared baking dish.

4. Drizzle with Olive Oil: Drizzle olive oil over the cod fillets, ensuring they are evenly coated.

5. Season with Herbs and Garlic: Sprinkle minced garlic, dried thyme, dried rosemary, dried oregano, salt, and pepper over the cod fillets. Ensure the herbs and garlic are distributed evenly.

6. Bake Cod: Bake in the preheated oven for approximately 15-20 minutes or until the cod is opaque and easily flakes with a fork.

7. Broil (Optional): If you desire a golden brown top, you can broil the cod for an additional 2-3 minutes, watching closely to prevent burning.

8. Garnish: Remove the baked cod from the oven. Garnish with freshly chopped parsley.

9. Serve: Plate the Baked Cod with Herbs and serve with lemon wedges on the side.

10. Enjoy Delight in the light and herby flavors of this perfectly baked cod.

Note: Adjust the herbs and seasonings to suit your taste preferences. Feel free to add a splash of white wine before baking for added depth of flavor.

Nutrition Information (per serving):

• Calories: 200 calories

• Protein: 25g

• Carbohydrates: 1g

• Sugars: 0g
• Fat: 12g

MISO-GLAZED MAHI-MAHI:

Meal Description: Indulge in the savory and umami flavors of Miso-Glazed Mahi-Mahi. This dish combines the rich taste of miso with the delicate and flaky texture of mahi-mahi. This simple and elegant recipe offers a delightful fusion of Japanese-inspired flavors that is sure to elevate your dining experience.

Ingredients:

For Miso Glaze:

- 1/4 cup white miso paste
- Two tablespoons of soy sauce
- One tablespoon of rice vinegar
- One tablespoon mirin (Japanese sweet rice wine)
- One tablespoon of honey or maple syrup
- One teaspoon of sesame oil
- Two cloves garlic, minced
- One teaspoon of fresh ginger, grated

For Mahi-Mahi:

- Four mahi-mahi fillets
- Sesame seeds and chopped green onions for garnish

• Lemon wedges for serving

Instructions:

1. Preheat Broiler: Preheat your oven's broiler.

2. Prepare Miso Glaze: In a bowl, whisk together white miso paste, soy sauce, rice vinegar, mirin, honey (or maple syrup), sesame oil, minced garlic, and grated ginger. Ensure the ingredients are well combined to create the miso glaze.

3. Marinate Mahi-Mahi: Place the mahi-mahi fillets in a shallow dish or a resealable plastic bag. Pour the miso glaze over the fillets, ensuring they are evenly coated. Marinate for at least 30 minutes in the refrigerator.

4. Broil Mahi-Mahi: Line a baking sheet with aluminum foil and lightly grease it. Place the marinated mahi-mahi fillets on the baking sheet. Broil for about 8-10 minutes, or until the fish is cooked through and flakes easily with a fork. Baste the fillets with the miso glaze halfway through cooking.

5. Garnish: Remove the mahi-mahi from the broiler. Garnish with sesame seeds and chopped green onions.

6. Serve: Plate the Miso-Glazed Mahi-Mahi and serve with lemon wedges on the side.

7. Enjoy the exquisite combination of the sweet and savory miso glaze with the succulent mahi-mahi.

Note: Adjust the sweetness and saltiness of the glaze to your taste preference. You can also grill the mahi-mahi if a broiler is not available.

Nutrition Information (per serving):

• Calories: 250 calories

• Protein: 35g

- Carbohydrates: 10g
- Sugars: 6g
- Fat: 8g

TUNA SALAD LETTUCE WRAPS:

Meal Description: Savor a light and satisfying meal with Tuna Salad Lettuce Wraps—a refreshing twist on the classic tuna salad, combining the goodness of tuna with the creaminess of Greek yogurt, all wrapped in crisp lettuce leaves. This low-carb and protein-packed dish is perfect for a quick, healthy lunch or snack.

Ingredients:

For Tuna Salad:

- Two cans (5 oz each) of tuna, drained

- 1/2 cup Greek yogurt

- One celery stalk, finely chopped

- 1/4 red onion, finely chopped

- One tablespoon of Dijon mustard

- One tablespoon of fresh lemon juice

- Salt and pepper to taste

- Fresh parsley, chopped, for garnish (optional)

For Lettuce Wraps:

- Large lettuce leaves (e.g., iceberg or butter lettuce)

- Cherry tomatoes, halved, for garnish

• Avocado slices, for garnish

Instructions:

1. Prepare Tuna Salad: In a mixing bowl, combine drained tuna, Greek yogurt, chopped celery, chopped red onion, Dijon mustard, fresh lemon juice, salt, and pepper. Mix until well combined.

2. Adjust Seasoning: Taste the tuna salad and adjust the seasoning, adding more salt, pepper, or lemon juice if needed.

3. Assemble Lettuce Wraps: Take large lettuce leaves, such as iceberg or butter lettuce, and spoon the tuna salad onto each leaf.

4. Garnish: Garnish the tuna salad with fresh parsley, cherry tomato halves, and slices of avocado.

5. Wrap and Serve: Fold the lettuce leaves around the tuna salad, creating wraps. Secure with toothpicks if desired.

6. Serve: Arrange the Tuna Salad Lettuce Wraps on a serving platter.

7. Enjoy these light and flavorful lettuce wraps as a delicious and healthy alternative to traditional sandwiches.

Note: For some heat, you can customize the tuna salad by adding ingredients like diced cucumber, capers, or a pinch of cayenne.

Nutrition Information (per serving):

• Calories: 200 calories

• Protein: 30g

• Carbohydrates: 8g

- Sugars: 3g
- Fat: 6g

SEARED HALIBUT WITH MANGO SALSA:

Meal Description: Elevate your dinner with the vibrant flavors of Seared Halibut topped with a refreshing Mango Salsa. This dish combines the delicate and flaky texture of halibut with the sweetness and tanginess of fresh mango salsa, creating a delightful and visually appealing meal.

Ingredients:

For Seared Halibut:

• Four halibut fillets

• Two tablespoons olive oil

• Salt and pepper to taste

• One teaspoon paprika (optional for additional flavor)

For Mango Salsa:

• One ripe mango, peeled, pitted, and diced

• 1/2 red bell pepper, finely chopped

• 1/4 red onion, finely chopped

• One jalapeño, seeded and finely chopped

• 1/4 cup fresh cilantro, chopped

- Juice of 1 lime

- Salt and pepper to taste

Instructions:

1. Prepare Mango Salsa: In a bowl, combine diced mango, chopped red bell pepper, finely chopped red onion, jalapeño, cilantro, lime juice, salt, and pepper. Mix well to create the mango salsa. Set aside.

2. Season Halibut: Pat the halibut fillets dry with a paper towel. Season both sides with salt, pepper, and paprika (if using).

3. Heat Olive Oil: Heat olive oil over medium-high heat in a skillet.

4. Sear Halibut: Place the halibut fillets in the hot skillet, skin side down if applicable. Sear for about 3-4 minutes on each side or until the halibut is golden brown and cooked through. The internal temperature should reach 145°F (63°C).

5. Serve: Transfer the seared halibut fillets to serving plates.

6. Top with Mango Salsa: Spoon the fresh Mango Salsa generously over each halibut fillet.

7. Garnish: Garnish with additional cilantro, if desired.

8. Serve Warm: Serve the Seared Halibut with Mango Salsa immediately while warm.

9. Enjoy: Enjoy the perfect balance of flavors and textures in each bite of this delightful and nutritious dish.

Note: You can serve this dish with a side of steamed rice, quinoa, or your favorite vegetables for a complete meal.

Nutrition Information (per serving):

- Calories: 250 calories
- Protein: 30g
- Carbohydrates: 15g
- Sugars: 10g
- Fat: 10g

SARDINE AND AVOCADO WRAP:

Meal Description: Experience a nutritious and flavorful combination with the Sardine and Avocado Wrap—a delicious assembly of mashed avocado, omega-3-rich sardines, and vibrant fresh veggies wrapped in a whole-grain tortilla. This quick and easy recipe perfectly balances creamy, savory, and crunchy elements for a satisfying and wholesome meal.

Ingredients:

• One can (about 3.75 oz) of sardines in olive oil, drained

• One ripe avocado, mashed

• One whole-grain wrap or tortilla

• 1/2 cup cherry tomatoes, halved

• 1/4 cup cucumber, thinly sliced

• 1/4 cup red bell pepper, thinly sliced

• Handful of mixed greens (e.g., arugula, spinach)

• Lemon juice for drizzling (optional)

• Salt and pepper to taste

Instructions:

1. Prepare Sardines: Drain the sardines and set aside.

2. Mash Avocado: In a bowl, mash the ripe avocado with a fork until smooth. Season with salt and pepper to taste.

3. Assemble Wrap: Lay the whole-grain wrap or tortilla on a flat surface. Spread the mashed avocado evenly over the wrap.

4. Add Sardines: Place the sardines evenly across the mashed avocado.

5. Layer Fresh Veggies: Add the halved cherry tomatoes, thinly sliced cucumber, and red bell pepper on top of the sardines.

6. Add Greens: Sprinkle a handful of mixed greens over the veggies.

7. Optional Drizzle: Drizzle a bit of lemon juice over the ingredients for a refreshing touch.

8. Wrap it Up: Fold the sides of the wrap and then roll it tightly, creating a secure wrap.

9. Slice and Serve: If preferred, diagonally slice the wrap in half for easier handling.

10. Enjoy: Enjoy the Sardine and Avocado Wrap immediately, savoring the combination of textures and flavors.

Note: For an extra kick, feel free to customize the wrap with additional ingredients like shredded carrots, red onion, or a dash of hot sauce.

Nutrition Information (approximate):

• Calories: 350 calories

• Protein: 20g

• Carbohydrates: 25g

- Sugars: 4g
- Fat: 20g

GRILLED MACKEREL WITH LEMON-HERB MARINADE:

Meal Description: Indulge in the robust flavors of Grilled Mackerel with Lemon-Herb Marinade—a dish that combines the rich taste of mackerel with the bright and zesty notes of lemon and herbs. The grilling process adds a smoky touch, creating a delightful seafood dish that's perfect for a light and satisfying meal.

Ingredients:

For Lemon-Herb Marinade:

• 1/4 cup olive oil

• Zest of 1 lemon

• Juice of 2 lemons

• Two cloves garlic, minced

• One tablespoon of fresh parsley chopped

• One tablespoon of fresh dill, chopped

• One teaspoon of fresh thyme leaves

• Salt and black pepper to taste

For Grilled Mackerel:

- Four mackerel fillets
- Lemon wedges for serving
- Fresh herbs for garnish (optional)

Instructions:

1. Prepare Lemon-Herb Marinade: In a bowl, whisk together olive oil, lemon zest, lemon juice, minced garlic, chopped parsley, chopped dill, fresh thyme leaves, salt, and black pepper. This creates the lemon-herb marinade.

2. Marinate Mackerel: Place the mackerel fillets in a shallow dish or a resealable plastic bag. Pour the lemon-herb marinade over the mackerel, ensuring each fillet is well-coated. Allow the mackerel to marinate in the refrigerator for at least 30 minutes.

3. Preheat Grill: Preheat your grill to medium-high heat.

4. Grill Mackerel: Remove the mackerel from the marinade and place them on the preheated grill. Grill for approximately 3-4 minutes per side or until the mackerel is cooked through and has an excellent grill mark.

5. Baste (Optional): Baste the mackerel with some of the remaining marinade during grilling for extra flavor.

6. Serve: Transfer the grilled mackerel fillets to a serving platter.

7. Garnish: Garnish with fresh herbs and lemon wedges.

8. Serve Warm: Serve the Grilled Mackerel with Lemon-Herb Marinade immediately while warm.

9. Enjoy: Relish this grilled mackerel's smoky, citrusy, and herby flavors.

Note: Serve the grilled mackerel with a side of steamed vegetables, quinoa, or a light salad for a well-balanced meal.

Nutrition Information (per serving):

- Calories: 250 calories

- Protein: 25g

- Carbohydrates: 2g

- Sugars: 1g

- Fat: 16g

CHAPTER SEVEN

Hydration Recipes

Cucumber and Mint Infused Water:

Beverage Description: Stay refreshed and hydrated with the delightful taste of Cucumber and Mint Infused Water. This simple and healthy beverage combines the crispness of cucumber with the cooling essence of fresh mint, creating a naturally flavored drink that's perfect for any time of day.

Ingredients:

• 1/2 cucumber, thinly sliced

• A handful of fresh mint leaves

• 1.5 liters (6 cups) cold water

• Ice cubes (optional)

• Lemon slices for garnish (optional)

Instructions:

1. Prepare Ingredients: Wash the cucumber thoroughly and slice it thinly. Rinse the fresh mint leaves.

2. Combine Cucumber and Mint: Combine the cucumber slices and fresh mint leaves in a large pitcher.

3. Add Cold Water: Pour cold water into the pitcher, covering the cucumber slices and mint leaves.

4. Refrigerate: Place the pitcher in the refrigerator to allow the flavors to infuse. Infuse for at least 2-4 hours or overnight for a more intense flavor.

5. Serve Over Ice (Optional): If desired, serve the infused water over ice cubes for a chilled experience.

6. Garnish (Optional): Garnish the infused water with additional cucumber slices or lemon slices for a decorative

touch.

7. Pour and Enjoy: Pour the Cucumber and Mint Infused Water into glasses and enjoy the refreshing taste.

Note: You can refill the pitcher with water a few times before replacing the cucumber and mint with fresh ingredients.

Variations:

• Experiment with other additions, such as lemon slices, lime slices, or a few crushed berries for additional flavor.

• Adjust the intensity of the infusion by letting it sit longer for a more pungent taste.

Benefits:

• Cucumber adds a subtle flavor and is hydrating.

• Mint provides a refreshing and cooling sensation.

• Infused water is a healthy alternative to sugary beverages.

WATERMELON BASIL COOLER:

Beverage Description: Quench your thirst and cool off with a refreshing Watermelon Basil Cooler. This hydrating summer drink combines watermelon's natural sweetness with fresh basil's aromatic essence. This simple blend is perfect for staying cool on hot days.

Ingredients:

• 4 cups seedless watermelon, cubed

• 1/4 cup fresh basil leaves

• 2 cups ice cubes

• One tablespoon of honey or agave syrup (optional, depending on watermelon sweetness)

• Fresh basil sprigs for garnish (optional)

• Watermelon slices for garnish (optional)

Instructions:

1. Prepare Ingredients: Cube the seedless watermelon and gather fresh basil leaves.

2. Blend Watermelon and Basil: Combine the cubed watermelon and fresh basil leaves in a blender.

3. Add Ice: Add the ice cubes to the blender. The ice will help create a chilled and slushy consistency.

4. Blend Until Smooth: Blend the ingredients until you achieve a smooth and slushy texture.

5. Taste and Sweeten (Optional): Taste the cooler and add honey or agave syrup if additional sweetness is desired. Blend again to incorporate.

6. Strain (Optional): If you prefer a smoother texture, you can strain the cooler using a fine mesh sieve to remove pulp.

7. Serve: Pour the Watermelon Basil Cooler into glasses.

8. Garnish (Optional): Garnish with fresh basil sprigs or watermelon slices for an extra touch.

9. Enjoy: Sip and enjoy the revitalizing taste of this hydrating summer drink.

Variations:

• Add a splash of lime juice for a citrusy kick.

• Experiment with other herbs like mint for a different flavor profile.

Benefits:

• Watermelon is hydrating and rich in vitamins A and C.

• Basil adds a refreshing herbal note and potential health benefits.

LEMON GINGER ICED TEA:

Beverage Description: Quench your thirst with the refreshing taste of Lemon Ginger Iced Tea. This refreshing and flavorful beverage combines the citrusy notes of lemon with ginger's warm, spicy essence. Brewed to perfection and served over ice, this iced tea is a delightful and hydrating choice, especially on warm days.

Ingredients:

• 4 cups water

• Four black tea bags

• One lemon, thinly sliced

• One tablespoon of fresh ginger, sliced or grated

• Ice cubes

• Fresh mint leaves for garnish (optional)

• Honey or sweetener of choice (optional)

Instructions:

1. Boil Water: Bring 4 cups of water to a boil in a saucepan.

2. Steep Tea Bags: Remove the saucepan from the heat and add the black tea bags. Depending on your desired strength, allow them to steep for 3-5 minutes.

3. Add Lemon and Ginger: While the tea is still hot, add the

thinly sliced lemon and fresh ginger to the saucepan. This allows the flavors to infuse as the tea cools.

4. Excellent Tea: Allow the tea to cool to room temperature. You can expedite this process by placing the saucepan in the refrigerator.

5. Strain (Optional): If you prefer a clear iced tea, you can strain out the lemon slices and ginger using a fine mesh sieve.

6. Refrigerate: Once cooled, refrigerate the tea until it is well chilled.

7. Serve Over Ice: Fill glasses with ice cubes and pour the chilled Lemon Ginger Iced Tea over the ice.

8. Sweeten (Optional): If desired, add honey or your preferred sweetener to the iced tea and stir until it's well combined.

9. Garnish (Optional): Garnish with fresh mint leaves for a burst of freshness.

10. Stir and Enjoy: Stir the iced tea, sit back, and enjoy the rejuvenating blend of lemon and ginger.

Variations:

• Green tea or herbal tea can be substituted for black tea for different flavor profiles.

• Experiment with other citrus fruits like orange or lime for a citrus-infused twist.

Benefits:

• Lemon provides vitamin C and a zesty flavor.

• Ginger adds warmth and potential digestive benefits.

COCONUT WATER SMOOTHIE:

Smoothie Description: Transport yourself to a tropical paradise with the Coconut Water Smoothie—a refreshing and hydrating blend of coconut water, pineapple, mango, and banana. Packed with tropical flavors and natural electrolytes, this smoothie is perfect for a revitalizing start to your day or a cooling treat in warmer weather.

Ingredients:

• 1 cup coconut water

• 1/2 cup pineapple chunks (fresh or frozen)

• 1/2 cup mango chunks (fresh or frozen)

• One ripe banana

• Ice cubes (optional for a colder texture)

• Unsweetened shredded coconut for garnish (optional)

Instructions:

1. Prepare Ingredients: If using fresh pineapple and mango, peel and chop them into chunks. Peel the banana.

2. Blend: In a blender, combine coconut water, pineapple chunks, mango chunks, and the ripe banana.

3. Add Ice (Optional): If you prefer a colder and icier texture, add a handful of ice cubes to the blender.

4. Blend Until Smooth: Blend the ingredients until you achieve a smooth and creamy consistency.

5. Taste and Adjust: Taste the smoothie and adjust the sweetness or thickness by adding more banana or coconut water if needed.

6. Pour into Glasses: Pour the Coconut Water Smoothie into glasses.

7. Garnish (Optional): Garnish with unsweetened shredded coconut for an extra tropical touch.

8. Serve: Serve immediately and enjoy the refreshing taste of this tropical coconut water smoothie.

Variations:

• Add a handful of spinach or kale for a green boost without compromising the tropical flavor.

• Include a scoop of protein powder for added protein.

Benefits:

• Coconut water is hydrating and a natural source of electrolytes.

• Pineapple and mango provide vitamins and antioxidants.

• Banana adds creaminess and natural sweetness.

SPARKLING BERRY WATER:

Beverage Description: Elevate your hydration experience with Sparkling Berry Water—a fizzy and refreshing drink that combines the effervescence of sparkling water with the vibrant flavors of mixed berries. This simple and hydrating concoction is perfect for those who crave a delightful and bubbly alternative to plain water.

Ingredients:

• 1 cup mixed berries (strawberries, blueberries, raspberries)

• 2 cups sparkling water

• Ice cubes

• Fresh mint leaves for garnish (optional)

• Lemon slices for garnish (optional)

Instructions:

1. Prepare Mixed Berries: Wash and hull the strawberries. If using larger berries, slice them into smaller pieces.

2. Muddle Berries (Optional): For a more intense berry flavor, gently muddle the mixed berries in the bottom of the glass using a muddler or the back of a spoon.

3. Add Sparkling Water: Place the mixed berries in a glass

and pour sparkling water over them. Adjust the quantity of sparkling water to achieve your desired level of fizziness.

4. Stir Gently: Give the Sparkling Berry Water a gentle stir to mix the berries and distribute the flavors.

5. Add Ice Cubes: Drop a few ice cubes into the glass to keep the drink cool.

6. Garnish (Optional): Garnish with fresh mint leaves and lemon slices for a burst of freshness.

7. Serve: Serve the Sparkling Berry Water immediately.

8. Enjoy: Sip and enjoy this sparkling berry-infused drink's crisp and fruity goodness.

Variations:

• Try different combinations of berries, such as blackberries, raspberries, or a splash of pomegranate seeds.

• Add a touch of sweetness with a drizzle of honey or agave syrup if desired.

Benefits:

• Berries are rich in antioxidants and vitamins.

• Sparkling water provides a bubbly and enjoyable drinking experience without added sugars.

BERRY-LIME SPARKLING WATER:

Beverage Description: Indulge in the vibrant fizz of Berry-Lime Sparkling Water. This refreshing and fruity beverage combines the sweetness of mixed berries with a splash of zesty lime, all in the effervescent embrace of sparkling water. This delightful drink is perfect for those who crave a burst of flavor without added sugars.

Ingredients:

• 1 cup mixed berries (strawberries, blueberries, raspberries)

• One tablespoon of fresh lime juice

• 2 cups sparkling water

• Ice cubes

• Fresh mint leaves for garnish (optional)

Instructions:

1. Prepare Mixed Berries: Wash and hull the strawberries. If using larger berries, slice them into smaller pieces.

2. Muddle Berries (Optional): For a more intense berry flavor, gently muddle the mixed berries in the bottom of the glass using a muddler or the back of a spoon.

3. Add Lime Juice: Squeeze fresh lime juice into the glass

with the mixed berries.

4. Add Sparkling Water: Pour sparkling water over the berries and lime juice. Adjust the quantity of sparkling water to achieve your preferred level of fizziness.

5. Stir Gently: Give the Berry-Lime Sparkling Water a gentle stir to mix the berries, lime, and sparkling water.

6. Add Ice Cubes: Drop a few ice cubes into the glass to keep the drink cool.

7. Garnish (Optional): Garnish with fresh mint leaves for an extra burst of freshness.

8. Serve: Serve the Berry-Lime Sparkling Water immediately.

9. Enjoy: Sip and enjoy the delightful combination of mixed berries, lime, and effervescent bubbles.

Variations:

• Experiment with different berries or add a splash of pomegranate juice for added depth of flavor.

• You can drizzle a bit of honey or agave syrup into the mix for a sweeter touch.

Benefits:

• Berries are rich in antioxidants and vitamins.

• Lime provides a zesty and citrusy kick.

• Sparkling water offers a bubbly and satisfying drinking experience without added sugars.

ICED HIBISCUS TEA WITH ORANGE SLICES:

Beverage Description: Experience the vibrant hues and refreshing taste of Iced Hibiscus Tea with Orange Slices—a delightful combination of tart hibiscus tea and the citrusy brightness of fresh orange slices. This chilled and visually appealing beverage is perfect for quenching your thirst with a burst of flavor on warm days.

Ingredients:

• Four hibiscus tea bags

• 4 cups hot water

• 1-2 tablespoons honey or sweetener of choice (optional)

• Orange slices for garnish

• Ice cubes

Instructions:

1. Brew Hibiscus Tea:

• Place hibiscus tea bags in a heatproof container.

• Pour hot water over the tea bags.

• Let the tea steep for 5-7 minutes or until it reaches your desired strength.

- Remove the tea bags.

1. Sweeten (Optional):

- Add honey or sweetener to the hot hibiscus tea and stir until dissolved.

- Adjust sweetness to your liking.

1. Cool and Chill:

- Allow the sweetened hibiscus tea to cool to room temperature.

- Once cooled, refrigerate the tea until it's well chilled.

1. Prepare Orange Slices:

- Slice fresh oranges into thin rounds or wedges.

1. Assemble Iced Tea:

- Fill glasses with ice cubes.

- Pour the chilled hibiscus tea over the ice.

1. Garnish:

- Garnish each glass with orange slices.

1. Stir and Serve:

- Give the iced hibiscus tea a gentle stir to incorporate the flavors.

- Serve immediately and enjoy the vibrant and cooling beverage.

Variations:

- Add a splash of sparkling water for a fizzy twist.

- Infuse the hibiscus tea with additional flavors like mint or ginger during brewing.

Benefits:

• Hibiscus tea is known for its potential health benefits, including antioxidants and aiding in digestion.

• Oranges provide vitamin C and a burst of citrusy flavor.

CONCLUSION

In conclusion, Lipedema poses a significant challenge to those affected, impacting not only their physical health but also their emotional well-being. This chronic condition demands a nuanced and comprehensive approach for effective management, recognizing the multifaceted nature of its symptoms and the individualized experiences of those living with it.

The RAD Diet for Lipedema emerges as a promising strategy, weaving together nutritional choices and lifestyle modifications to address the unique aspects of this condition. By acknowledging the role of inflammation, lymphatic dysfunction, and hormonal influences on fat distribution, the RAD Diet offers a holistic framework that goes beyond conventional weight loss methods. It seeks to empower individuals by providing them with practical tools to navigate the complexities of living with lipedema.

One of the RAD Diet's strengths is its adaptability, recognizing the diversity of experiences among individuals with lipedema. The diet acknowledges that there is no one-size-fits-all solution and emphasizes flexibility, allowing for personalized adjustments to suit individual needs and preferences.

Furthermore, the RAD Diet not only addresses the physical aspects of lipedema but also considers the psychological impact of living with a chronic condition. Fostering a positive and supportive dietary environment aims to enhance the overall quality of life for those affected, providing a sense of control and empowerment.

As our understanding of lipedema continues to evolve, the RAD Diet stands as a beacon of hope for those seeking comprehensive and tailored approaches to manage this condition. Ongoing research, coupled with increased awareness and advocacy, holds the potential to refine further and expand the strategies available for individuals with lipedema.